Build Big Arms
Revised Edition

Written and Published by Bill Pearl
Edited by George and Tuesday Coates
Layout and Illustrations by Richard R. Thornley Jr.

Bill Pearl
P.O. Box 1080
Phoenix, Oregon 97535
Email: support@billpearl.com
Website: www.billpearl.com

ISBN-13: 978-1-938855-08-5

Notice of Rights

Medical Disclaimer - See Your Doctor

Most people may do all of the exercises found in this book with no ill effects. However, if certain movements cause discomfort they should be eliminated. See your doctor and get the doctor's approval on the total fitness program.

Table of Contents

Chapter 1

Introduction

Big arms fascinate people regardless of their knowledge or interest in exercise or sports. Even though they do not openly admit their desire to obtain large arms... the desire is still there.

To satisfy the demand for such information, Bill Pearl, the world's best built man, has written this first in a series of books on exercise. No one is better qualified to instruct you than the man who has done the job himself and has helped his students gain far beyond what they had hoped for in physical development. Bill Pearl has won every major award for physical excellence. Among his titles are Mr. America, Mr. USA, and Mr. Universe. He has toured the world giving demonstrations and lectures on the subject of exercise. He has designed a complete book for developing your arms at the local gym, YMCA, or in your own home. These three courses are the ones he personally uses in training to build his mighty 20 1/2 inch arms. These are the exercises he feels have done the job.

Bill's arms are the envy of millions and he has continued to improve them through the years. Let his experience help you. Be wise, follow the programs to the letter and do not attempt to improvise. If you work hard, you'll obtain the big arms you desire

Good Luck!
Leo Stern

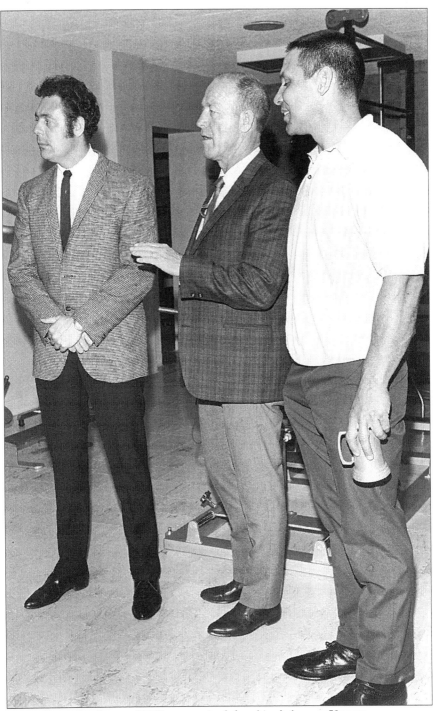

George Coates, Leo Stern and Bill have remained close friends for over 50 years.

Chapter 2

Building Big Arms

Big arms dominate the thoughts of all bodybuilders. In view of this fact, I will try to assist you in acquiring bigger and better arms. On the following pages, you will find the three main courses I have personally used for some time and which I feel is the answer to many of the problems of building better biceps and triceps.

After many years of concentrated effort, I have designed and completed this book, which I am sure will help you increase your arm size considerably. Please sit down and read it thoroughly before starting the courses. You will eliminate several problems that might arise later.

Do not feel that since I have listed three sets of eight repetitions for an exercise that you will promote faster growth by increasing the number of sets to five or six each. You can over work the muscle, just as you can fail to work them enough. There is a normal balance and the number of sets and repetitions listed are ideal for these particular programs.

The sets and repetitions are as I do them. Realizing that this will not be suitable for all of you, as some have been exercising regularly for just a short period of time and others have been training for many years, the courses are listed in two groups. #1 is the advanced group and #2 the intermediate. With limited training, it is not advisable to try to work in the same group as those who have spent a number of years training. Decide for yourself which category you belong in.

Please follow the sequence listed and do not alter the arrangement in the program in any way. It is my desire to help you and this I cannot do unless you follow the instructions precisely and... Trust in me.

Concentration while doing an exercise is of extreme importance in getting the maximum work from the muscle. Also, try to maintain a proper mental attitude towards your workouts and approach each workout session with a purpose in mind to improve.

Best of Luck,
Bill Pearl

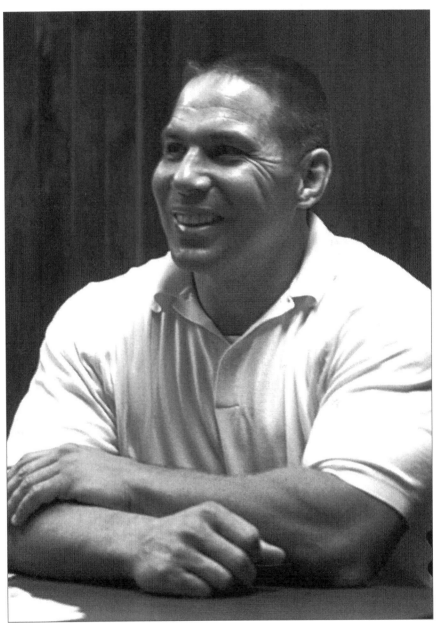
Bill Pearl smiling after a good days work.

Chapter 3

How to Use this Book

If a person is interested in weight training for more than basic conditioning, it is imperative that he study each illustration and description before attempting a new exercise. Progress definitely can be deterred if an exercise is done incorrectly.

Many exercises can be accomplished with the exact same motion but will affect different areas of a muscle by the angle at which the exercise is performed. For example: an exercise done on a flat bench, or an incline bench, will put different emphasis on the same muscle even though the same motion, weight and equipment are used.

It is therefore necessary to perform exercises from as many different angles that are reasonable and to use as many variations that are reasonable to develop a fully matured muscular physique.

On the following pages, highly accurate drawings appear that will enable you to see the pieces of equipment used to perform each exercise and the style used for each movement. Each exercise includes the proper name of the exercise, the muscle group most affected, "degree of difficulty" information, and a written description of how the exercise should be done.

The "degree of difficulty" information appearing below each exercise heading will give you at a glance what exercise may be suited for your present physical condition.

NOTE: It is not necessarily true that an exercise considered "easy" may not be just as effective as one considered "hard". Any exercise can be made more or less difficult, depending on the weight used or the effort put forth.

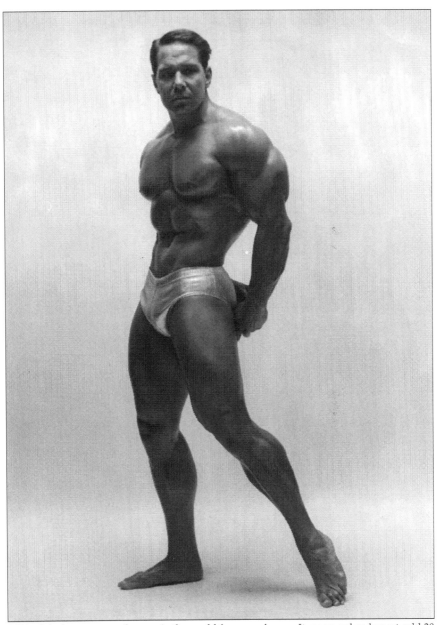

Bill had the largest muscular arm in the world for several years. It measured an honest cold 20 3/8 inches at a bodyweight of 218 pounds.

Chapter 4

Equipment Needed

Equipment needed to perform the exercises in this training guide.

- Barbell
- Dumbbells
- Flat Bench
- Incline Bench
- Dip Stand
- Lat Machine

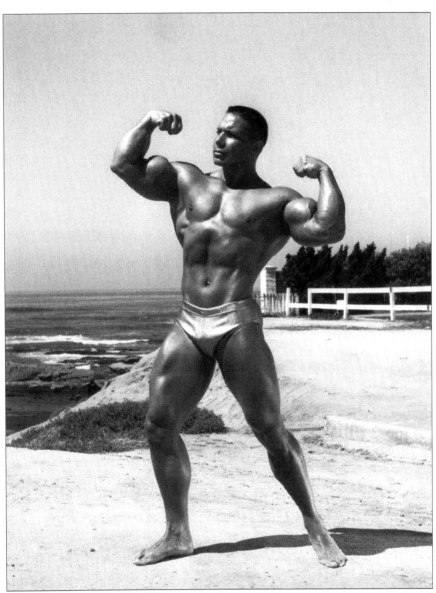

At this stage of Pearl's bodybuilding career, he had changed to a lacto-ovo-vegetarian diet and was still able to maintain his massive size.

Chapter 5

Course One

EXERCISES:

1. Standing Close Grip Triceps Press Down on Lat Machine	3 sets of 10
2. Lying Supine Medium Grip Barbell Triceps Curl and Press	3 sets of 8
3. Dips	3 sets of 10-12
4. Standing Medium Grip Barbell Curl	3 sets of 8
5. Incline Dumbbell Curl	3 sets of 8
6. Standing Dumbbell Curl	3 sets of 8

- Follow this course of exercises for a six week period
- Do Three Workouts per Week

Before getting into the Big Arms Program, there are a few rules that should be followed. These rules are very important to your building large, well-shaped muscular arms.

First, you must do all the exercises as strictly as possible. Do not cheat on any of the movements. Try to get a complete extension and contraction on each movement and handle a poundage that will enable you to do this. Concentrate on the area that you are working on and train at a speed that will keep that area warm. With a little experimenting on your part, you will be able to find the pace best suited for you. Last, but not least, keep a daily record of the weights you are using for each exercise and be sure to train in a progressive manner.

Weight Progression

The system that I have found to be ideal for myself is the following, for example take the triceps exercise with pulley, you start with 50 lbs. and do 3 sets of the required repetitions. I would do this same weight for the first three workouts. On my fourth workout I would do 2 sets with the 50 lbs. and 1 set with the 60 lbs. On my fifth workout I would do 1 set with 50 lbs. and 2 sets with the 60 lbs. On the sixth workout I would do all my sets with 60 lbs. From there on advance the weight continuing to do 3 sets with the same weight like the seventh workout 3 sets with 65 lbs. and the tenth workout with 75 lbs. Now remember the poundage mentioned is merely for example. You will of course use the poundage in proportion to your ability and strength, just be sure to start fairly light so that you can do all the exercises right.

In regard to the balance of your workout, I would suggest that you continue to do at least 2 sets for each body part. For instance continue to do 2 sets of chest, 2 sets of thigh, etc. Do not neglect the rest of your body just for the sake of arm development.

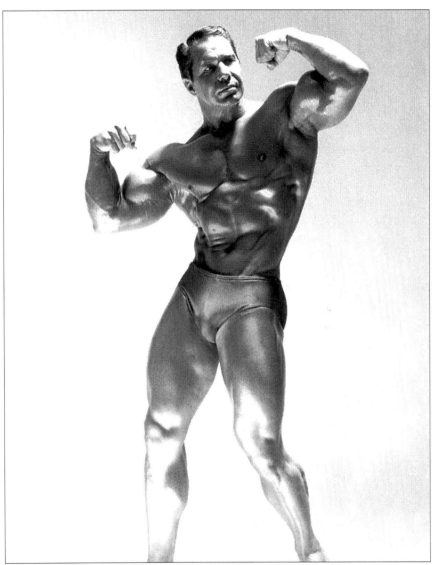

From any angle or pose Bill assumes, size, symmetry, proportions were all uniform. A gift from God and hard work.

STANDING CLOSE GRIP TRICEPS PRESS DOWN ON LAT MACHINE

Muscle Group: Outer triceps
Degree of Difficulty: Intermediate

Stand erect in front of a let machine with your feet about sixteen inches apart and your back straight. Grasp the let machine bar with both hands using a palms down grip about eight inches apart. Bring your upper arms to your sides and keep them there throughout the exercise. Your forearms and biceps should be touching as you inhale and then press the bar down in a semicircular motion to arm's length. Return to starting position using a similar path, in a controlled manner, and exhale. Be sure to keep tension on your triceps while pressing down and returning to starting position

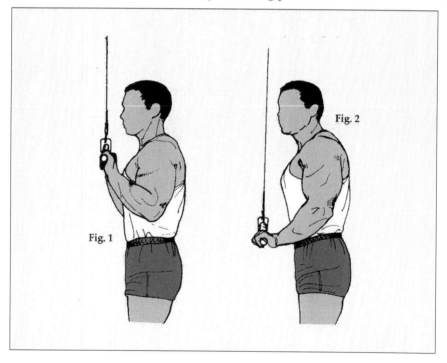

Fig. 2

Fig. 1

LYING SUPINE MEDIUM GRIP BARBELL TRICEPS CURL AND PRESS

Muscle Group: Triceps
Degree of Difficulty: Intermediate

Hold a barbell with both hands using a palms down grip about fourteen inches apart. Lie on a flat bench with your head on the bench keeping your chin pointing upward. Press the barbell to arm's length keeping it in line with your shoulders. Inhale and lower the barbell down in a semicircular motion by bending your arms at the elbows but keeping your upper arms vertical. The barbell should be lowered to your chin and your forearms and biceps should touch. Now pull the barbell over to your chest and place it just below the nipples of your pectorals. Press the bar back to arm's length keeping your elbows in close to cause the triceps muscles to do the work and exhale.

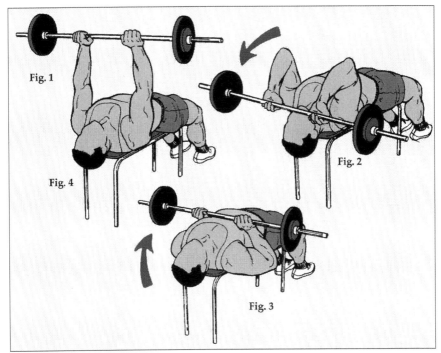

Fig. 1

Fig. 2

Fig. 3

Fig. 4

DIPS

Muscle Group: Pectorals and triceps
Degree of Difficulty: Difficult

Use a set of parallel bars or a regular dip stand for this exercise. Position yourself on the bars so you are held erect by your arms but able to drop to a low position without having your feet touch the floor. Keep your elbows into your sides as much as possible while lowering your body downward by bending your arms. You should continue downward until your forearms and biceps come together. Pause a short time and then press yourself back to arm's length forcing a lock out of the elbows thereby contracting the triceps and pectoral muscles. Do not let your body swing back and forth during this exercise. With a little practice and concentration, it will be very easy for you to control the body position. Inhale as you lower yourself and exhale as you push yourself back to starting position.

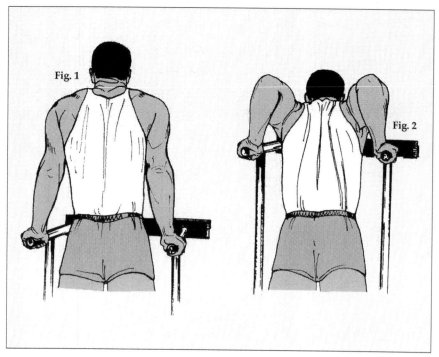

STANDING MEDIUM GRIP BARBELL CURL

Muscle Group: Biceps
Degree of Difficulty: Intermediate
Hold a barbell with both hands using a palms-up grip about eighteen inches apart. Stand erect with your feet about sixteen inches apart. With the barbell at arm's length against your upper thighs, inhale and curl the bar up to the height of your shoulders keeping your back straight, legs and hips locked out. As you are lowering the bar back to starting position, do so in a controlled manner causing the biceps to resist the weight as much as possible. Exhale as you return to starting position.

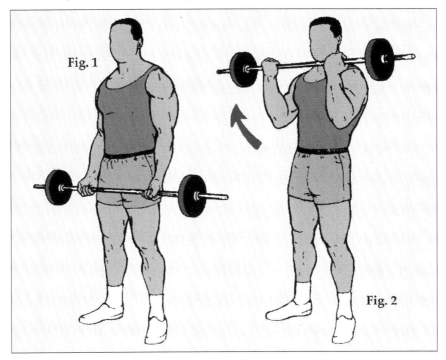

Fig. 1

Fig. 2

INCLINE DUMBBELL CURL

Muscle Group: Biceps
Degree of Difficulty: Intermediate

Hold a dumbbell in each hand and lie back on an incline bench with your head up and feet on the footpads. With the dumbbells hanging at arm's length at your sides, with your palms in, inhale and curl the dumbbells up to the height of your shoulders. As you commence the curl and the dumbbells are past your thighs, then turn your palms-up and keep them in this position throughout the exercise until you are lowering the weights and again near your upper thighs before turning your palms in again and exhaling. Keep your upper arms in close to your sides and concentrate or your biceps raising and lowering the weights.

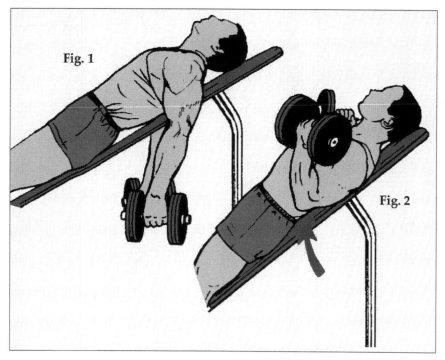

STANDING DUMBBELL CURL

Muscle Group: Biceps
Degree of Difficulty: Intermediate

Hold a dumbbell in each hand and stand erect with your feet about sixteen inches apart. Keep your back straight, head up, and hips and legs locked out. With the dumbbells hanging at arm's length at your sides, with your palms in, inhale and curl the dumbbells up to the height of your shoulders. As you commence the curl and the dumbbells are past your thighs, then turn your palms-up and keep them in this position throughout the exercise until you are lowering the weights and again near your upper thighs before turning your palms in again and exhaling. Keep your upper arms in close to your sides and concentrate on your biceps raising and lowering the weights.

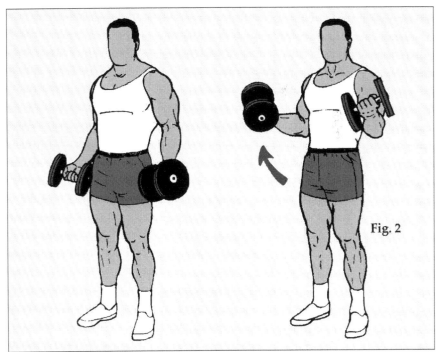

Fig. 2

Chapter 6

Course Two

EXERCISES:

1. Seated Dumbbell Curl	3 sets of 8
2. Incline Medium Grip Barbell Triceps Curl	4 sets of 8
3. Lying Supine Dumbbell Curl	3 sets of 8
4. Lying Supine Two Dumbbell Triceps Curl	4 sets of 8
5. Seated Concentrated Dumbbell Curl	3 sets of 8
6. Standing Dumbbell Triceps Curl	4 sets of 8

- Follow this course of exercises for a five week period
- Do Three Workouts per Week

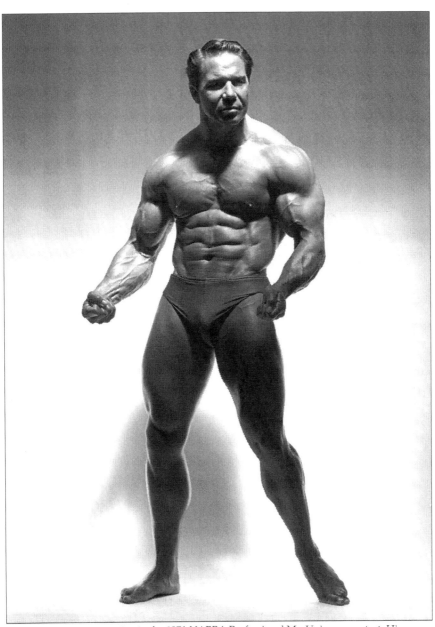

Pearl just prior to competing in the 1971 NABBA Professional Mr. Universe contest. His bodyweight was 242 pounds.

SEATED DUMBBELL CURL

Muscle Group: Biceps
Degree of Difficulty: Intermediate

Hold a dumbbell in each hand and sit at the end of a flat bench with your back straight, head up and feet planted firmly on the floor. With the dumbbells hanging at arm's length at your sides, with your palms in, inhale and curl the dumbbells up to the height of your shoulders. As you commence the curl and the dumbbells are past your thighs, then turn your palms-up and keep them in this position throughout the exercise until you are lowering the weights and again near your upper thighs before turning your palms in again and exhaling. Keep your upper arms in close to your sides and concentrate on your biceps raising and lowering the weights.

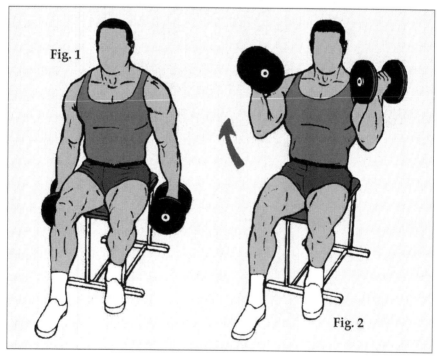

Fig. 1

Fig. 2

INCLINE MEDIUM GRIP BARBELL TRICEPS CURL

Muscle Group: Triceps
Degree of Difficulty: Intermediate

Hold a barbell with both hands using a palms down grip about fourteen inches apart. Lie back on an incline bench and press the barbell overhead to arm's length. Inhale and lower the weight down behind your head in a semi-circular motion by bending your arms at the elbows but keeping your upper arms vertical throughout the exercise. Keep your head up and off the bench to allow the barbell to go between your head and the bench. The barbell should be lowered until your forearms and biceps touch. Press the barbell back to starting position using the same path and exhale. Be sure to keep your upper arms as close to the sides of your head as possible during the exercise.

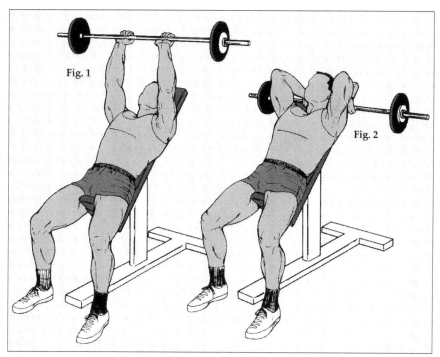

Fig. 1

Fig. 2

LYING SUPINE DUMBBELL CURL

Muscle Group: Biceps

Degree of Difficulty: Intermediate

Hold a dumbbell in each hand and lie in a supine position on a flat bench with your head up and legs to the sides of the bench for better balance. With the dumbbells hanging at arm's length straight down, with your palms in, inhale and curl the dumbbells up to the height of your shoulders. As you commence the curl turn your palms-up and keep them in this position throughout the exercise until you are lowering the weights and again near the end of the curl and then turn the palms in. Keep your upper arms in close to your sides and concentrate on your biceps raising and lowering the weights

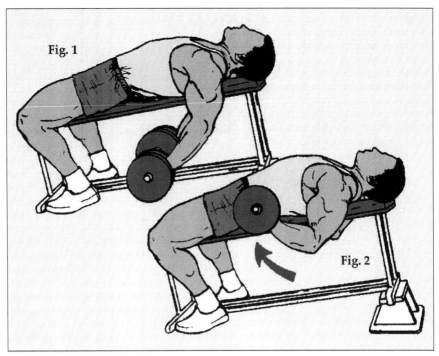

LYING SUPINE TWO DUMBBELL TRICEPS CURL

Muscle Group: Triceps
Degree of Difficulty: Intermediate

Lie on a flat bench. Hold a dumbbell in each hand and press them to arm's length keeping them in line with your shoulders. Inhale and lower both dumbbells straight down in a semicircular motion by bending your arms at the elbows but keeping your upper arms vertical throughout the exercise. The dumbbells should be lowered until your forearms and biceps touch. Press the dumbbells back to starting position using the same path and exhale.

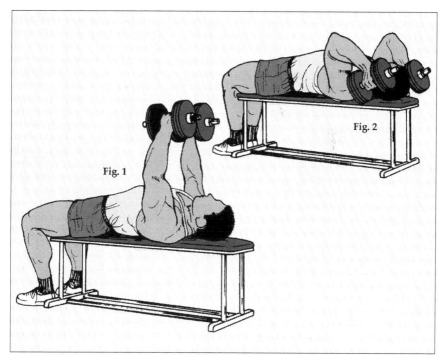

Fig. 1

Fig. 2

SEATED CONCENTRATED DUMBBELL CURL

Muscle Group: Biceps

Degree of Difficulty: Intermediate

Grasp a dumbbell in your right hand and sit on a bench with your feet about twenty-four inches apart. Position the dumbbell in front of you hanging at arm's length between your legs with a palms-up grip. Bend slightly at the waist and place your left hand on your left knee to help support your upper body. Rest your upper right arm against your inner right thigh about four inches above your knee. Inhale and curl the dumbbell upward in a semicircular motion by bending your arm at the elbow and keeping your upper arm vertical with the floor. Continue the curl until your biceps and forearm are touching. At the top position the dumbbell should be shoulder height. Return to starting position using a similar motion and exhale. Do the prescribed number of repetitions with your right arm and then change positions doing the same number of repetitions with your left arm.

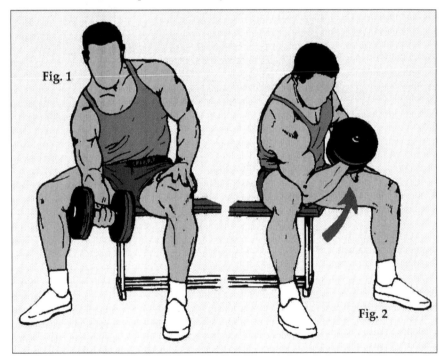

Fig. 1

Fig. 2

STANDING DUMBBELL TRICEPS CURL

Muscle Group: Triceps
Degree of Difficulty: Difficult

Grasp one dumbbell with both hands and raise it overhead to arm's length, vertical with the floor. As you are raising the dumbbell rotate your hands up and over until the top plates are resting in the palms of your hands while your thumbs remain around the handle. Stand erect with your back straight, head up and feet about sixteen inches apart. Keep your upper arms in close to the sides of your head during the exercise. Inhale and lower the dumbbell behind your head in a semicircular motion until your forearms and biceps touch. Return the weight to starting position using a similar path and exhale.

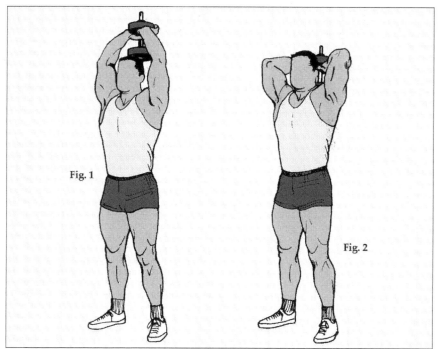

Fig. 1

Fig. 2

Chapter 7

Course Three

EXERCISES:

1. Standing Medium Grip Barbell Triceps Curl	4 sets of 8
2. Lying Supine Medium Grip Barbell Triceps Curl to Forehead	4 sets of 8
3. Standing Dumbbell Triceps Curl	4 sets of 8
4. Incline Dumbbell Curl	3 sets of 8
5. Incline Inner Biceps Curl	3 sets of 8
6. Seated Concentrated Dumbbell Curl	3 sets of 15

- Follow this course of exercises for a four week period
- Do Three Workouts per Week

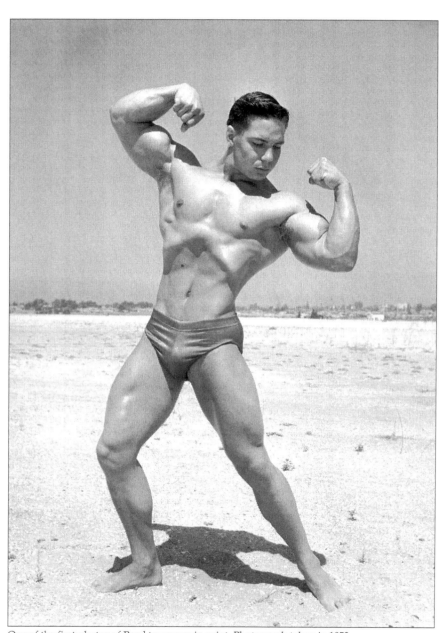

One of the first photos of Pearl to appear in print. Photograph taken in 1952.

STANDING MEDIUM GRIP BARBELL TRICEPS CURL

Muscle Group: Triceps
Degree of Difficulty: Intermediate

Hold a barbell with both hands using a palms down grip about fourteen inches apart. Stand erect with your back straight, head up and feet about sixteen inches apart. Press the barbell overhead to arm's length. Inhale and lower the weight down behind your head in a semicircular motion by bending your arms at the elbows but keeping your upper arms vertical throughout the exercise. The barbell should be lowered until your forearms and biceps touch. Press the barbell back to starting position using the same path and exhale. Be sure to keep your upper arms as close to the sides of your head as possible during the exercise.

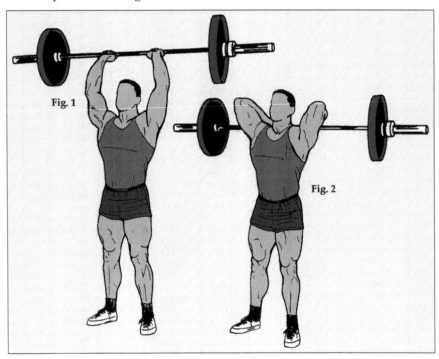

Fig. 1

Fig. 2

LYING SUPINE MEDIUM GRIP BARBELL TRICEPS CURL TO FOREHEAD

Muscle Group: Triceps
Degree of Difficulty: Intermediate

Hold a barbell with both hands using a palms down grip about fourteen inches apart. Lie on a flat bench keeping your head on the bench. Press the barbell to arm's length keeping it in line with your shoulders. Inhale and lower the barbell down in a semicircular motion by bending your arms at your elbows but keeping your upper arms vertical throughout the exercise. The barbell should be lowered to your forehead and your forearms and biceps should touch. Press the barbell back to starting position using the same path and exhale.

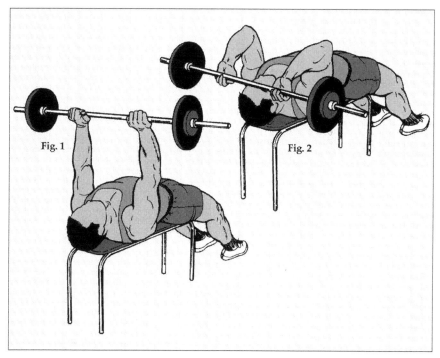

Fig. 1   Fig. 2

STANDING DUMBBELL TRICEPS CURL

Muscle Group: Triceps
Degree of Difficulty: Difficult

Grasp one dumbbell with both hands and raise it overhead to arm's length, vertical with the floor. As you are raising the dumbbell rotate your hands up and over until the top plates are resting in the palms of your hands while your thumbs remain around the handle. Stand erect with your back straight, head up and feet about sixteen inches apart. Keep your upper arms in close to the sides of your head during the exercise. Inhale and lower the dumbbell behind your head in a semicircular motion until your forearms and biceps touch. Return the weight to starting position using a similar path and exhale.

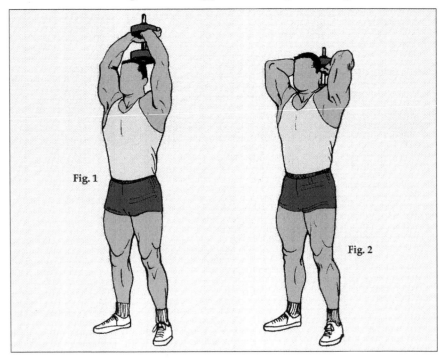

Fig. 1

Fig. 2

INCLINE DUMBBELL CURL

Muscle Group: Biceps
Degree of Difficulty: Intermediate

Hold a dumbbell in each hand and lie back on an incline bench with your head up and feet on the footpads. With the dumbbells hanging at arm's length at your sides, with your palms in, inhale and curl the dumbbells up to the height of your shoulders. As you commence the curl and the dumbbells are past your thighs, then turn your palms-up and keep them in this position throughout the exercise until you are lowering the weights and again near your upper thighs before turning your palms in again and exhaling. Keep your upper arms in close to your sides and concentrate or your biceps raising and lowering the weights.

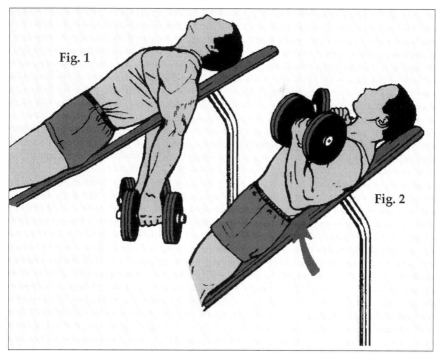

INCLINE INNER BICEPS CURL

Muscle Group: Inner biceps
Degree of Difficulty: Difficult

Hold a dumbbell in each hand and lie back on an incline bench with your
head down and feet on the footpads. With the dumbbells at arm's length
hanging at your sides and your palms facing in, inhale and curl the dumbbells up as you turn your palms-up. Curl the weights outward and up keeping your forearms in line with your outer deltoids. Continue the curl until
the dumbbells are at shoulder height and to the sides of your deltoids. Lower
the weights back to starting position using the same path of resistance and
exhale.

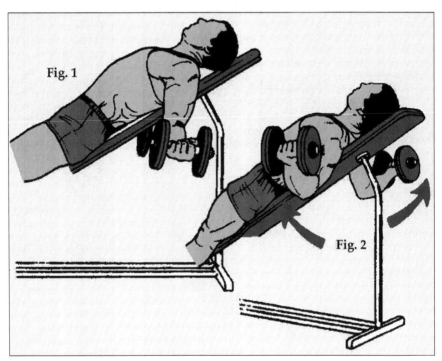

Fig. 1

Fig. 2

SEATED CONCENTRATED DUMBBELL CURL

Muscle Group: Biceps
Degree of Difficulty: Intermediate

Grasp a dumbbell in your right hand and sit on a bench with your feet about twenty-four inches apart. Position the dumbbell in front of you hanging at arm's length between your legs with a palms-up grip. Bend slightly at the waist and place your left hand on your left knee to help support your upper body. Rest your upper right arm against your inner right thigh about four inches above your knee. Inhale and curl the dumbbell upward in a semicircular motion by bending your arm at the elbow and keeping your upper arm vertical with the floor. Continue the curl until your biceps and forearm are touching. At the top position the dumbbell should be shoulder height. Return to starting position using a similar motion and exhale. Do the prescribed number of repetitions with your right arm and then change positions doing the same number of repetitions with your left arm.

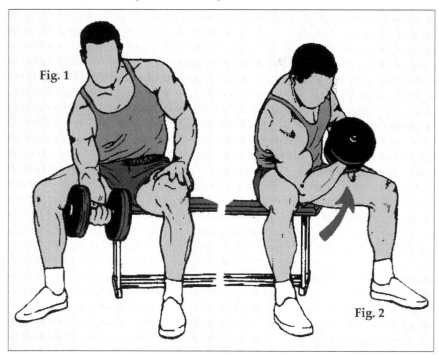

Fig. 1

Fig. 2

Chapter 8

Triceps Pump or Extension

The object of this exercise is to keep the triceps pumped and full of blood while working the biceps. I suggest that you do not try this method of working the arms on any of the other programs because it is too much for the average person. Also you will not get full benefit from it.

After having worked the triceps as illustrated in Course #3, and started on the biceps exercise, this exercise may be used as a means of keeping the triceps pumped during the biceps work.

I have found the following workout is best: Complete two sets of the dumbbell curls on incline and then do a triceps pump. Do the final set of dumbbell curls on incline and one set of the incline inner biceps curls and another pumping movement. In other words, after every two sets of biceps curls, do a pumping movement. This will be carried out throughout the entire biceps workout.

The proper way to do the triceps pump is as follows: Place yourself in starting position that is shown in figure 1 on the next page, with your head lowered. Obtain an object that is about 25 inches off the floor that will enable you to get a good hand grip and extend out far enough. With your back and buttocks in a straight position, lower yourself to the position shown in figure 2. Notice that you lower yourself until your head is between the hands and the forearms and biceps are compressed. The back and buttocks are still in straight position. From the position in figure 2, use the triceps to raise body back to starting position. Again, it is very important to keep elbows in as much as possible and put all the strain on the triceps.

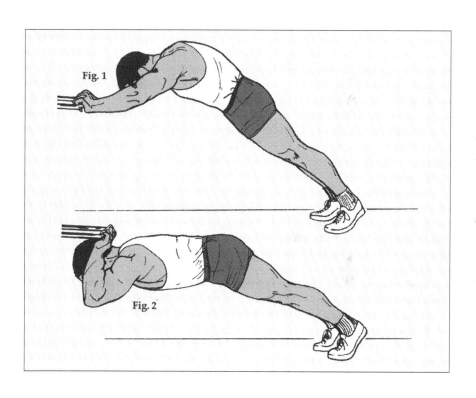

Fig. 1

Fig. 2

37

Chapter 9

Intermediate Sets

The following sets are designed for intermediate trainers, and should be used in place of those listed opposite the exercises for each course. However, the exercises remain the same... only the sets are reduced.

EXERCISES FOR COURSE ONE:

1. Standing Close Grip Triceps Press Down on Lat Machine	2 sets of 8
2. Lying Supine Medium Grip Barbell Triceps Curl and Press	2 sets of 8
3. Dips	2 sets of 10-12
4. Standing Medium Grip Barbell Curl	2 sets of 8
5. Incline Dumbbell Curl	2 sets of 8
6. Standing Dumbbell Curl	1 set of 8

EXERCISES FOR COURSE TWO:

1. Seated Dumbbell Curl	2 sets of 8
2. Incline Medium Grip Barbell Triceps Curl	2 sets of 8
3. Lying Supine Dumbbell Curl	2 sets of 8
4. Lying Supine Two Dumbbell Triceps Curl	2 sets of 8
5. Seated Concentrated Dumbbell Curl	2 sets of 8
6. Standing Dumbbell Triceps Curl	2 sets of 8

EXERCISES FOR COURSE THREE:

1. Standing Medium Grip Barbell Triceps Curl	2 sets of 8
2. Lying Supine Medium Grip Barbell Triceps Curl to Forehead	2 sets of 8
3. Standing Dumbbell Triceps Curl	2 sets of 8
4. Incline Dumbbell Curl	2 sets of 8
5. Incline Inner Biceps Curl	2 sets of 8
6. Seated Concentrated Dumbbell Curl	1 sets of 15

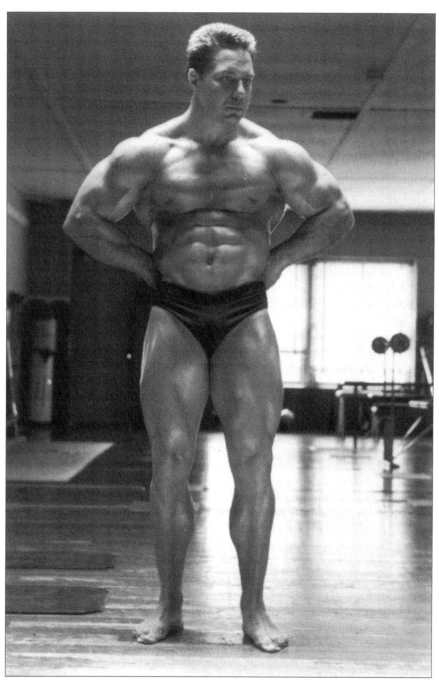

A photo of Bill, as he prepared to guest pose for the 1956 Mr. Hawaii contest

This page has been intentionally left blank.

Made in the USA
San Bernardino, CA
27 July 2018